GUT FRIENDLY RAMADAN GUIDE

DISCOVER HOW TO NURTURE YOUR BODY DURING RAMADAN AND BEYOND IN A GUT HEALTHY WAY

TAHIRA ISMAIL

Copyright © 2024 by Tahira Ismail - All rights reserved.

No part of this publication may be reproduced, stored, or transmitted in any form or by any means, electronic, mechanical, photocopying, recording, scanning, or otherwise, without written permission from the publisher. It is illegal to copy this book, post it to a website, or distribute it by any other means without permission.

Tahira Ismail asserts the moral right to be identified as the author of this work. Tahira Ismail has no responsibility for the persistence or accuracy of URLs for external or third-party Internet Websites referred to in this publication and does not guarantee that any content on such websites is, or will remain, accurate or appropriate.

Designations used by companies to distinguish their products are often claimed as trademarks. All brand names and product names used in this book and on its cover are trade names, service marks, trademarks, and registered trademarks of their respective owners. The publishers and the book are not associated with any product or vendor mentioned in this book. None of the companies referenced within the book have endorsed the book.

Disclaimer Notice: Please note the information contained within this document is for educational purposes only. All effort has been executed to present accurate, up-to-date, and reliable, complete information. No warranties of any kind are declared or implied. Readers acknowledge that the author is not engaging in the rendering of legal, financial, medical, or professional advice. The content within this book has been derived from various sources. Please consult a licensed professional before attempting any techniques outlined in this book.

By reading this document, the reader agrees that under no circumstances is the author responsible for any losses, direct or indirect, which are incurred as a result of the use of the information contained within this document, including, but not limited to, — errors, omissions, or inaccuracies.

First edition

Dedicated to my father and family for their unwavering support and endless encouragement. Thank you to Saliha Nazir and Zaynab Bokhari for their editing prowess. Thank you to Maymuna for being my number-one fan.

Contents

Introduction	VII
1. Why Gut Health?	1
2. Immune System	5
3. Nutrition	9
4. Stress	17
5. Environment & Toxicity	21
6. Medications & Antibiotics	27
7. Sleep	29
8. Physical Activity	33
9. Hydration	37
10. Putting It All Together	39
11. Optimizing Ramadan With Gut Health	43
12. Don'ts - Foods to Avoid	49
13. Do's - What To Eat & Drink	57
14. Avoid Overeating	67
Final Thoughts	69
Bonus Recipes	71
Glossary	83

Resources

INTRODUCTION

Gut health is essential in every season of life, including Ramadan. When you take care of your overall health—including your gut health—then going through spiritual acts becomes much more fulfilling and rewarding as your concentration can be focused away from your personal health concerns.

Your gut is known as the body's 'second brain,' and keeping it healthy is critical for the health of the rest of your body. Even if you don't have noticeable gut issues, your gut contains organisms that promote healing, positive mental health, and balancing hormones. Understanding why it's important will motivate you to take steps to have a healthy gut and, in turn, become a healthier version of yourself. On top of that, I hope, if you don't already, you will start planning and organizing to get the most out of your days and nights in Ramadan. It only comes around once a year, and we do not know if we will be there for the next, so it's vital to treat it like our last!

Ramadan is a month that about 2 billion people look forward to every year. It is filled with anticipation for children and adults alike. During Ramadan, Muslims fast from dawn to sunset for 29 to 30 days. Since the Islamic calendar is lunar, the start and end of it move forward approximately 11 days each year. So, over a period of 33 years, Ramadan's appearance will be from summer to spring to winter and then to fall. If you live in a relatively similar region during that time, you will experience Ramadan with the shortest and longest days of the year. The easiest days and the most challenging.

O believers! Fasting is prescribed for you - as it was prescribed for those before you - so perhaps you will become mindful 'of God'. Al-Baqarah 183

Ramadan is not only a time to abstain from food and drink but also a time for self-reflection, refraining from bad deeds (more than usual), increasing good deeds and charity, reading the Quran, performing extra prayers, and not wasting time. To accomplish this to the best of your ability, some effort and planning must take place. Just as with anything, you can't expect to go into the month without any plans or changes and expect to emerge as a different person.

Taking care of our body is not just something we do a week or month before Ramadan. Rather, we must focus on this throughout the year so that all holidays and seasons can be fruitful and enjoyed.

MY STORY

In my younger years, eating healthy was not high on my priority list. I ate for two reasons: first, to satisfy my hunger, and second, for enjoyment. And I ate heartily. The extra calories had no effect on me, and at that time, being healthy equaled being thin—and thin was something I was. It never fazed me that my urgent need for a bathroom soon after eating wasn't normal. In hindsight, I was likely thin due to leaky gut or intestinal permeability and the fact that I wasn't digesting most of what I ate. As a result, not only was I thin, but I was malnourished, which eventually would have led to illnesses and diseases if the problem had not been rectified. Alhamdulillah, I realized what I was doing to myself before it was too late.

1

Why Gut Health?

Before we get into simple ways to plan for a better Ramadan, let's briefly discuss your gut. After all, only when you begin to understand why it's essential to take care of your gut health in all seasons of life will you begin to take positive action.

First of all, what is your gut? The gut is a term used to describe the gastrointestinal tract, also commonly called your digestive system. The three terms are often used interchangeably. Entering through your mouth, food begins its digestive journey by being chewed—releasing enzymes and breaking down food to safely travel down the esophagus and into the stomach. The stomach plays a vital role in further digestion later on (ensuring that it can safely travel through the other organs). It further breaks down the food by adding in acid and more enzymes, turning it into mush or a thick paste. After the stomach has finished its job, the food continues to move through the gut and into the small intestine (which, ironically, is over 20 feet long in a grown adult!). The pancreas and liver kick into action and release more enzymes and bile, further breaking the food down. These enzymes are needed to break down proteins, carbs, and fats. Throughout this process, your body extracts nutrients from the food and uses them for energy or stores excess for later use.

The gut holds a series of roles, including hosting much of your immune system and serving as a communication hub for various bodily functions. From there, the food travels to the large intestine (also known as the colon and is up to 7 feet long, although it is much wider in diameter than the small intestine). Once food enters the large intestine, the focus is producing waste, which is then excreted through the rectum. When discussing the gut, we are mainly talking about the stomach, small intestine, and colon, but it's important to understand the other organs' roles.

Unfortunately, many people assume that they don't need to pay special attention to the health of their gut, particularly if they don't suffer from bloating, constipation, or stomach aches. Gut health is vastly undervalued by the majority of people today.

However, while you may not feel symptoms similar to stomach aches or bloating, it doesn't mean your stomach is healthy. The body often responds by producing a series of secondary symptoms when it is not functioning at its best. In fact, nearly all illnesses and diseases begin in the gut, which is why it is so important to focus on gut health.

Let's look at something as seemingly simple as acne. Many people who suffer from skin conditions such as acne or psoriasis have an imbalance in their gut microbiota; and, while it could be any host of gut conditions, often these are traced back to a condition known as leaky gut.

Leaky gut is when the tight junctions in your intestine loosen up and let food particles and toxins escape into parts of your body through the bloodstream and into areas where they should not be. As a result, you become prone to all sorts of illnesses and autoimmune disorders, and further gut complications. The effects on your body could be damaging to short and long-term health.

Other conditions that are directly related to gut health include (but are not limited to):

- Alzheimer's Disease
- Anxiety
- Autism Spectrum Disorders
- Autoimmune Diseases
- Cardiovascular Disease
- Celiac Disease
- Chronic Fatigue Syndrome (CFS)
- Chronic Kidney Disease
- Chronic Urticaria (Hives)
- Colorectal Cancer
- Constipation
- Depression
- Diarrhea
- Eczema
- Food Allergies

- Gallstones
- Gastroesophageal Reflux Disease (GERD)
- Inflammatory Bowel Disease (IBD)
- Irritable Bowel Syndrome (IBS)
- Leaky Gut Syndrome
- Metabolic Syndrome
- Migraines
- Mood swings
- Non-Alcoholic Fatty Liver Disease (NAFLD)
- Obesity
- Parkinson's Disease
- Psoriasis
- Small Intestinal Bacterial Overgrowth (SIBO)
- Type 2 Diabetes

Your gut health is no joke; you must take care of it.

When considering the health of your gut, you must take a step back and evaluate the health of your whole body: you have to look at the whole picture, not just an individual detail.

2

IMMUNE SYSTEM

We 'perfectly' ordained 'its development'. How excellent are We in doing so! Al-Mursalat 23

The gut contains a variety of organisms, more collectively known as the microbiome: viruses, bacteria, fungi, and other microbes. There are good and bad variations of these, and you want as many good ones in your gut as possible.

Most diseases that begin in the gut are a result of an imbalanced microbiome. While your immune system is found in many parts of your body, the majority of it — approximately 70% — is located in your gut. When your gut is healthy, you are well on your way to having a healthy immune system. When your gut is damaged, chances are you have a weakened immune system. You can't have one without the other!

The immune system builds and develops from birth, taking about a decade to develop into a fully functional, healthy gut system. As babies and children are exposed to the natural environment, they begin to build their immune systems. The gut's immune system is typically the strongest throughout the late teenage years and all the way to about retirement age. During this time, our immune systems become fully active and functioning, increasing in strength every time we are exposed to viruses, bacteria, fungi, and other microbes. Exposure to minor illnesses, colds, and cases of flu is actually very good for building our immune system! And, when you are continually exposed to different things but seldom get sick, well, that's a sign that your immune system is in great shape. When sickness, even something as simple as a cold, goes around, we often notice that the very young and the very old are prone to getting the sickest. This all stems back to the strength of their immune system and gut health.

Your immune system is primarily made up of two parts: the innate immune system and the adaptive immune system. The innate system is the first to act by preventing pathogens (an organism that causes disease) from multiplying or spreading. The adaptive immune system has a much more delayed response but is more specialized and relies on antibodies to produce a customized response against the pathogen. A robust immune system has both a strong innate and adaptive immune system.

Whether you often catch colds and bugs or simply have bad skin, then it's time to look at your gut health and what could be compromising it. Your gut health and how you treat it is the most crucial factor when dealing with your overall health.

RABIYA'S STORY

Rabiya came to me with a complaint of bloating and constipation. On top of that, she and her family were prone to catching every cold that went around. After our first meeting, I realized that based on her lifestyle, diet, and medical history, most likely, her and her family's gut health was very weak. We immediately went to work on removing problematic foods, adding in nourishing foods, and improving aspects of their lifestyle, all with the intention of repairing their gut health. Thankfully, the bloating and constipation subsided. About a year later, I ran into Rabiya at the grocery store. I asked her how she was doing and if she was still getting ill frequently. She stared at me momentarily and suddenly realized that she hadn't had a cold since fixing her gut! She had embraced her new normal and completely forgot how she used to feel. Her immune system was doing its job well now that her gut was fully functioning.

3

NUTRITION

O humanity! Eat from what is lawful and good on the earth and do not follow Satan's footsteps. He is truly your sworn enemy. Al-Baqarah 168

Your body is highly receptive to the environment, and as a result, when it is treated right, the gut can become very healthy. Conversely, when your body is not treated well, it begins to show symptoms, indicating that the gut microbiome is imbalanced. And the number one way to mistreat or heal your gut microbiome is through nutrition: foods, drinks, and supplements.

The Standard American Diet, also known as SAD, is one of the biggest problems affecting the health of North Americans today. The average person consumes foods filled with processed ingredients or food lacking nutritional value, which only provides empty calories. Many of these foods are loaded with artificial colors, flavors, preservatives, additives, chemicals, and more. Many of these have been linked to cancer, hyperactivity, and other deadly diseases.

However, processed foods are just the beginning of the problem. Many types of food, whether packaged or not, have alarmingly high amounts of refined sugar. While the fat portion of a meal or snack is usually accused of causing weight gain, we know for sure that it's the added sugar that makes you put on the extra pounds. From yogurt to pasta sauces, the number of tablespoons in a single container can be shocking. Take, for example, the very popular tomato sauce brand *Prego*. At the time of writing, a half-cup of sauce (equivalent to about one serving) has 10 grams or roughly three teaspoons of sugar! And many organic and 'healthy' versions are comparable to this. Canned soups, granola bars, low-fat yogurt, cereal and protein bars, and many brands of non-dairy milk—all supposedly 'healthier' options — are infamous for the amount of sugar they contain. Processed foods are slowly killing the average person.

Not only has sugar caused obesity to rise, but it's also the leading cause of diabetes. The story of sugar is extensive, but it causes much more than fat and obesity. Many pathogens and cancers feed on sugar, causing diseases to multiply quickly and flourish, taking over your body at alarming rates. Even the brain responds to sugar—in a similar way it does to cocaine! People don't realize it, but sugar is highly addictive and needs to be limited.

As stated earlier, the gut microbiome comprises viruses, bacteria, and fungi. While that may sound frightening, in reality, there are good and bad types of organisms. For a gut to be healthy, the good needs to outweigh the bad to keep it in check. You need the good kinds of bacteria and fungi in your gut. Processed foods, and particularly sugar, are food for harmful organisms.

As a result, these cause bad organisms to flourish, and as you might be assuming, hence begins a series of poor health. And, as also stated earlier, most diseases and conditions begin in the gut!

Okay, so most people know that sugar, processed foods, fried foods, and similar types of food are not conducive to good health. Even if one indulges in them more often than they should, there is an understanding that it's not healthy food. You must realize that this could be wreaking havoc on your body and have lasting long-term consequences. You must be conscious of everything you put into your body. You are what you eat!

So, say you don't indulge often but still suffer from auto-immune conditions and other health issues, major or minor. What could be the cause?

Not all food is equal, and not all bodies react to food in the same way. Depending on your gut microbiome and how it developed through childhood, your gut may or may not be able to handle certain foods. Even some healthy foods might not be suitable for you and may cause damage to your gut. A sore gut or throwing up is often a first reaction (and a severe one), but often, we also must listen to other symptoms: acne, fatigue, arthritis flare-ups, etc. These can all be reactions to the food you are consuming.

Food sensitivities are another big issue that usually escapes many people's radars. Unlike food allergies, whose effects are typically felt fairly quickly, food sensitivities don't necessarily show their effects right away. It could be a few hours or even days.

So, how does someone determine if their gut is healthy or needs some help? Listen to your body. Start keeping a food journal and tracking your food and any symptoms you may have, then you are more likely to begin to understand your body, its likes, and dislikes, and can make changes accordingly. It's time to get out of auto-pilot and deeply listen to your body when you eat and in the hours after you've consumed food. And ask yourself questions such as:

- How am I feeling physically today? How is this different from yesterday, last week, or last month?

- What is my emotional state like today? Can this be traced back to a particular event or circumstance, or is it 'just my mood'?

- How are my bowel movements? Are they regular, or are they more reminiscent of diarrhea or constipation?

- Is something I'm eating making me sick? Sometimes, it's eating too much; sometimes, it's not eating enough. Perhaps your body loves avocado, but maybe it can't tolerate more than half an avocado. Some people can't eat any, while others have absolutely no issue with it at all.

The food you eat has varied nutritional value. Fruits and vegetables contain various vitamins and minerals needed for your body to function well. However, they also serve as food for your gut microbiome. After all, the 100 trillion microorganisms need to be fed! The better the quality of your food, the more nutritional value it has. Eating a bag of chips versus a piece of fruit or some vegetables will have vastly different effects on the body and the health of your gut, even if they have the same number of calories. The chips will essentially feed the harmful organisms, while the fruits and vegetables feed the good. Everything you eat affects your gut and your overall health.

Even fruits and vegetables vary in nutrition. Some are known to be superfoods because of the large quantity of nutritional value they provide or because they have unique nutrients that many diets lack; adding the right foods to your diet can drastically improve your gut microbiome.

Many of these are readily accessible at your local grocery store and at reasonable prices.

- Avocado: This rich green food is packed with monounsaturated fats, vitamins, and minerals. Not only is it good for your gut, but also for brain and heart health.

- Beans and lentils: These are excellent sources of protein (beneficial for maintaining energy when fasting), fiber, and important vitamins and minerals.

- Berries (blueberries, raspberries, strawberries): Berries are filled with a range of antioxidants and vitamins.

- Broccoli (and other cruciferous vegetables): They contain vitamins C and K, insoluble fiber, and various antioxidants.

- Chia seeds: High in omega-3 fatty acids, fiber, and protein, these can easily be added to smoothies, yogurt, and soups.

- Cocoa (dark chocolate): Contains much-needed flavonoids that have antioxidant properties.

- Eggs: A complete protein source with various vitamins and minerals critical to gut health.

- Garlic: Known for its immune-boosting properties and potential cardiovascular benefits, it can be easily added to many different types of main courses.

- Greek yogurt: This is an excellent source of protein, probiotics, and calcium and can easily be added to a meal or used as a snack.

- Green tea: An underestimated drink that you need to add to your diet because it is rich in antioxidants, notably catechins, which help prevent chronic diseases.

- Leafy greens (kale, lettuce, spinach, swiss chard): You need these in your diet as they are an excellent source of vitamins, minerals, and antioxidants for your gut.

- Mushrooms: The more unique the variety, the more nutrients and immune-boosting properties they have.

- Nuts: These are important sources of healthy fats, protein, vitamins and minerals.

- Pumpkin seeds: Often underestimated and not included in the diet, these are high in magnesium, iron, zinc, and protein.

- Quinoa: This is a complete protein source with a good balance of all essential amino acids and can easily be substituted for pasta or rice.

- Salmon: An excellent source of quality protein rich in omega-3 fatty acids and vitamin D.

- Sweet Potatoes: Another frequently underestimated vegetable rich in vitamins A and C, fiber, and antioxidants.

- Tomatoes: A family favorite, this vegetable is rich in antioxidants, including lycopene, and can be used as the base for many sauces.

- Turmeric: A powerful spice that contains curcumin, a powerful anti-inflammatory compound.

Finally, always shop for non-GMO (genetically modified organisms) and organic foods as these will have the highest nutritional value but also lack chemicals that destroy the gut microbiome. More on this later.

When shopping at the grocery store, stick to the outside aisles as they contain fruits, vegetables, seafood, and meats. This is also where the foods with the most nutritional value can be found.

Noura's STORY

Noura was suffering from low energy and back acne. Acne she had for over ten years. She wanted to eat healthy but was confused about the conflicting information she was running into. With new diets and food trends continually popping up, she needed clarification on where to start. Together, Noura and I focused on nutritious foods (and learning why she needed a wide range of fruits and vegetables), ensuring that she cleaned up her diet, reduced her sugar consumption, and found healthier snacks. Within a few months, her back acne had cleared up, and her energy was soaring!

4

STRESS

When we study our body closely, we realize what a captivating and interesting topic of study it is. And many people don't realize how much stress can damage it. The environment around us can have a lasting effect on our physical, mental, and emotional health. The environment refers to the physical aspect of it, the atmosphere around us, the situations we put ourselves in, and how we treat ourselves.

One key aspect of our gut health is our relationship with stress. In fact, stress can have nearly the same negative effect on our body as other aspects of how we treat it, including nutrition. Many different factors can cause distress and imbalance in the gut organisms, which in turn causes illnesses and diseases.

Stress wreaks havoc on your body in multiple ways. Even if you eat the most nutritious meals, stress will prevent your gut from absorbing all those excellent nutrients. While some degree of stress is normal, and your body is designed to be able to handle it, continuous, high-intensity stress is a serious problem. It will activate stress hormones in your body, such as cortisol and adrenaline. Stress hormones are not meant to be easily activated and can cause particular conditions such as insulin resistance, which in turn can lead to diabetes, obesity, and even cardiovascular disease. Chronic stress can negatively affect every system in the body, including the gastrointestinal system. Other conditions that would be activated include:

- Raised inflammatory response.

- The corruption of cells in the body.

- The limitation of the body's ability to heal itself.

Finally, stress can also affect your immune system's memory and slow its response to pathogens.

To determine if you are stressed, you can ask yourself the following questions:

- Am I suffering from headaches, tension headaches, muscle tension, or chronic fatigue?

- Do I suffer from lack of sleep, difficulty sleeping, or falling asleep?

- Do I have unexplained weight or eating issues?

- Do I have unexplained emotional difficulties or cognitive disabilities?

- Am I satisfied with my life and circumstances?

Your mind and gut are interconnected and affect each other interchangeably. For many people, stress can trigger digestive problems such as, but not limited to, diarrhea and bloating. If someone is constantly having diarrhea, then that means they are not absorbing the nutrients from their food and are essentially flushing them down the toilet. Once you are nutritionally deficient, this can lead to further illnesses, ailments, and diseases.

So, it's essential to get stress under control with stress management strategies; whether from self-care or therapy, find what works best for you, but remember Allah first. Everything is in His hands, and reaching out to Him is of the utmost importance and value.

Allahuma rahmataka 'arjoo falaa takilnee 'ilaa nafsee tarfata 'aynin, wa 'aslih lee sha'nee kullahu, laa'illaha 'illaa 'Anta

Translation

O Allah, I hope for Your mercy. Do not leave me to myself even for the blinking of an eye. Correct all of my affairs for me. There is none worthy of worship but You.

After *dhikr* and *dua*, here are some of my favorite ways to reduce and manage stress:

- Journaling
- Breathing exercises
- Time management
- Avoiding sugar, caffeine, and other stimulants
- Exercising
- Socializing
- Counseling

- Mindfulness and visualization

NADIA'S STORY

Nadia was doing everything right. Well, almost everything. She ate plenty of vegetables and fruits, limited her grains, and avoided sugar, processed foods, and vegetable oils. But she still felt miserable. Random bouts of diarrhea would attack her digestive system, often without little warning. It got so bad that she no longer desired to leave the home and was afraid to eat anything when she did have to leave the house. After our first appointment, I realized that I wasn't the person she primarily needed help from; she needed a therapist. What Nadia hadn't realized was that the stress she was experiencing was causing her digestive system to speed up and expel whatever was in her. After speaking with a therapist, learning and applying stress-reducing techniques, and working on her relationship with Allah, her gut was much more at ease. Then, in tandem with her therapist, Nadia and I worked on nutrition to build up and strengthen her body again.

5

ENVIRONMENT & TOXICITY

A serious gut disruptor is your environment and toxin level. Over the last century, the number of chemicals we have become exposed to has risen exponentially. Modest estimates put the number of chemicals we are exposed to at 700,000, whereas a more accurate estimate is thought to be around 2.1 million. From cleaning products to the fabric of your clothing, your body must constantly filter thousands of toxins to keep your body healthy.

With millions of toxins and chemicals worldwide, we are continually subjected to their ill side effects. And different chemicals can cause a variety of damage to the body. Consuming or being exposed to chemicals can cause the healthy variety of bacteria in your gut to be depleted or severely damaged, leading to all sorts of complications throughout the body. For example, many chemicals are obesogens, which cause you to gain weight or prevent you from losing it.

Perhaps someone is eating right and exercising, and their stress is under control, but they can't seem to lose the extra pounds that are stubbornly clinging to them. What could be going on? It could very likely be that their toxic load is too high for their body to process. And if you have many of these obesogens in your body, you won't be able to lose weight because the fat is shielding you from the dangerous chemicals. The fat wraps itself around the chemical, and until you stop taking in the chemicals, you won't be able to lose that excess fat. This is just one way that toxins affect your health.

Chemicals can cause skin conditions, respiratory illnesses, allergies, cancer, and other deadly conditions. They essentially affect every system in your body, but their first place of target is typically the gut.

Chemicals can be everywhere, from your shower curtain, pots and pans, chemical cleaners, food, cosmetics, and personal care products. That is exposure to thousands of chemicals, many of which have *not* been tested by governments and health organizations for their safety with neither short nor long-term safety in mind.

So, it's time to take note of what toxins are in your life and take a step-by-step approach to removing them. Toxins place an incredible amount of stress on the gut and the body in general. Your body was designed to be able to flush out the toxins, but the number of toxins we expose it to makes it difficult for it to thoroughly and accurately flush out continually. We must take responsibility for our health; to do that, we must remove toxins from our homes and body. It will have a lasting positive impact on our short-term and long-term health.

To remove toxins in your home environment, do an inventory of what you have and start replacing it in a manner that works for you and your budget. The sooner you remove the toxins from your life, the quicker you can remove them from your body and start healing.

The following areas are regions of the home with a high level of toxins that can easily be reduced by replacing key items.

Kitchen:

Check the kitchen for Teflon pots and pans and plastic containing BPA or other chemicals.

- Use organic and non-GMO foods
- Opt for food stored in glass rather than tin
- Avoid non-stick pots and pans (stick to glass, ceramic, and stainless steel, not aluminum, when possible)
- Replace plastics with glass
- Replace plastic cutting boards with glass or high-quality wood
- Avoid plastic wrap
- Avoid using aluminum foil

Cleaning Products:

Are your cleaners filled with toxic chemicals, or are they plant-based with gentle ingredients?

- Use organic and natural cleaners
- Replace air fresheners with essential oil diffusers
- Use natural laundry detergents or make your own
- Don't use fabric softeners or dryer sheets that rely on synthetic fragrances or wax
- Regularly replace air and furnace filters

Personal Products:

Personal products should be on the top of your list of items to replace as they often have lengthy contact with your skin. Are you spraying and slathering yourself with poisons?

- Use natural cosmetics, soaps, shampoos, and conditioners
- Use non-scented and natural hygiene products

Also, it's not just these products we need to be concerned with; check your plastic items; things with strong scents (such as shower curtains and cheap toys) are probably not that good for you. Strong smells or odors contain a plethora of chemicals that slowly damage your body.

Unfortunately, many of these toxic products look deceptively pleasing. We see beautiful things and want to surround ourselves with them or use them to our benefit. Sadly, these shiny, pretty things are slowly destroying us.

Say, 'O Prophet,' "Good (tayyib things, deeds, beliefs, foods, etc.) and evil (Al-Khabith things deeds, beliefs, foods, etc.) are not equal, though you may be dazzled by the abundance of evil. So be mindful of God, O people of reason, so you may be successful." Al-Ma'idah 100

For more information, please see my first book, **The Secrets of Household Toxins**, which takes a deep dive into where chemicals may be lurking in your house, their harmful effects, how to remove them, and their safe alternatives.

SALMA'S STORY

Salma was struggling to breathe as pain radiated throughout her body. Her kids took notice and began to panic, unsure of what to do. As time went on and the symptoms got worse, they decided it was time to take her to the emergency room at their local hospital. When Salma's husband arrived home, he took one look at her and asked if she had been doing some deep cleaning. Salma admitted she had been. Salma's husband then reminded her that her body reacted like this whenever she deep cleaned. After visiting me, Salma began to understand the harm the toxic chemicals were having. Once we came up with alternative natural cleaners, her deep cleaning sessions became uneventful!

6

MEDICATIONS & ANTIBIOTICS

While we are discussing chemicals, let's also discuss medications and antibiotics. While I will definitely say there is a time and place for medicine and antibiotics, and I do not recommend going off of them without consulting your doctor, it is known that both of them are over-prescribed and can cause a multitude of negative side effects that can cause long-term damage to various organs.

Medication and antibiotics may be helpful in certain situations, but they aren't without side effects. Antibiotics are used to treat bacterial infections, and while they kill off or prevent the growth of harmful bacteria, unfortunately, they also kill the good and much-needed bacteria in our gut needed for a healthy gut. Many gut conditions stem from over-antibiotic use or even from one antibiotic treatment. It's essential only to take them when absolutely necessary. In addition, medications can cause diarrhea, heartburn, constipation, and more.

If you are currently taking medications and antibiotics and would like to remove them eventually, you must make health your number one priority. Maintaining a healthy weight, regularly exercising, and sleeping well are all key to removing these horrific toxins from your life.

Even if you have conditions requiring medications for the rest of your life, you can still improve your symptoms by caring for your gut health. The overall improvement of your life and condition can be traced back to your gut. So take the next step, do the next thing that can change your life: get your gut healthy.

Remember, medicine is not a magic pill. If possible, try improving your nutrition and lifestyle habits first. You might be pleasantly surprised!

"There is no disease that Allah has created, except that He also has created its treatment." [Al-Bukhari].

MARYAM'S STORY

As a child, Maryam had multiple ear infections. At the time, it wasn't known that her regular milk consumption was the cause of them. She never slowed down drinking milk, and every time another ear infection showed up, she went through another bout of antibiotics. However, the repeated prescriptions of antibiotics caused severe and ongoing damage to her gut microbiome—there was a severe lack of gut microbiota left in her intestines. As an adult, Maryam had various gut imbalances that caused her daily pain and irregular bowel movements, which resulted in a weakened immune system. It wasn't until she put a special focus on improving her gut health through diet as well as by adding in healing foods, supplements, and probiotics that she was finally able to live without daily pain.

7

SLEEP

He is the One Who has made the night for you as a cover, and 'made' sleep for resting, and the day for rising.
Al-Furqan 47

Let's briefly talk about sleep. We all know we need sleep, but why? Our bodies are designed to be able to handle everyday problems, stressors, illnesses, and other things that pop up. One of our natural healing mechanisms is sleep. While we sleep, our body has the time to repair itself from all those everyday problems, remove toxins, release hormones, and so on.

When we do not get enough sleep, it will cause stress on our entire body, not just the brain. Therefore, it will also negatively affect our gut microbiome. Studies show that just 2 days of poor sleep will alter your gut microbes, cause inflammation, and will activate your stress hormones. So, if your sleep is lacking, then you need to figure out why and work on it.

Ask yourself questions such as:

- Do you need to improve your sleep hygiene?

- Are you exposed to a lot of blue light right before bed?

- Is your mind active with the day's happenings or stressful news you were exposed to?

- How many hours of sleep do you get every day?

As you try to improve your sleep quality, here are some tips to help you prepare for bed and lengthen the time and quality of your sleep.

- Avoid difficult or emotional topics later in the day. If you have something on your mind that you are afraid you will forget about, write it down.

- Avoid screen time (laptops, phones, tablets, etc.) one hour before bed.

- Turn overhead lights off and use floor or table lights one hour before bed.

- Avoid eating late at night or before bed.

- Come up with a relaxing evening routine, such as drinking herbal tea, taking a bath, listening to the Quran, and reading books.

Eating late in the day is another factor in losing sleep that may not have occurred to you. Late-night eating can cause bloating and digestive discomfort that can disrupt sleep. It's best to finish eating at least a few hours before bedtime to ensure proper digestion and comfort. In addition, when your body needs to digest food as you sleep, it focuses on just that rather than fixing and repairing aspects of your physical health. This includes the production and release of *cytokines*, critical for your immune system and how it responds to pathogens. Another important aspect of sleep is the release of growth hormones, which are critical for repairing damaged cells.

SAFIA'S STORY

Safia's life was plagued by constant gas and acid reflux, leading to sleepless nights, which affected every aspect of her life, including her weak immune system. Prescription medications offered only temporary relief before the symptoms came back with full force. Determined to regain control, we examined her diet, identified fast and fried foods as culprits, and made significant nutritional improvements. By addressing her sleep habits, including eliminating late-night eating and blue light exposure, her symptoms faded. With better sleep and improved nutrition, she transformed into a well-rested, energized person, experiencing enhanced daily focus and endurance.

8

Physical Activity

What role does physical activity play in our gut health? We all know that some sort of physical activity is good for our overall health. We don't need to be running marathons or going to a gym, but it's essential to be active in whatever capacity you can, ranging from walking (an underrated activity), team sports, or even just working in your garden and everything in between.

Movement is absolutely vital for our gut health. Regular exercise increases blood flow in our digestive system, which helps keep us regular, meaning less constipation and less bloating. Physical activity has also been shown to increase the beneficial bacteria in our gut microbiome. More variety of beneficial bacteria means better gut health.

The gut has millions of microorganisms, and the healthy ones thrive and promote diversity in the microbiome when exercise is introduced and utilized. As you exercise and the diversity in your gut increases, you'll improve your gut's ability to move food through the intestines, limiting the damaging effects of stationary food on your gut and digestive system.

Likewise, your immune system is also positively affected when exercising — which, as previously discussed, is mainly found in the gut. Finally, physical activity can positively impact the gut by reducing the gaps in your intestines, a condition known as gut permeability or leaky gut.

So again, choose an activity that is within your capacity and that you enjoy. It could be team sports, lifting weights, doing workouts from an app, or just walking or working in the garden. All movement is beneficial. Start today by taking a short walk and slowly build yourself up to about 10,000 steps a day. Remember, you don't need to do all your exercising in one go - even bite-size, five-minute intervals several times throughout the day are sufficient.

Our beloved Prophet (May Peace and Blessings Be Upon Him) said: "The strong believer is better and more beloved to Allah than the weak believer, while there is good in both" [Muslim].

This strength refers to both physical strength and strength of faith. So we are encouraged to exercise and we get bonus points for archery, swimming, and horse riding, which the Prophet (*May Peace and Blessings Be Upon Him*) had recommended.

Before we move to the next chapter, don't forget to get moving after eating a meal or snack. Even a five-minute walk around the block or your home will help keep your gut in tip-top shape and flush out the toxins from your body. And yes, physical activity is important when fasting, just not as intensely.

Omar's STORY

Omar's health took a back seat until he realized his constipation was far from normal. Research revealed his diet and water intake were decent, but his sedentary lifestyle was the culprit. Adding a daily half-hour walk sparked change. Suddenly, he discovered he was having bowel movements after his walk. Soon, he upgraded to a 3km run, incorporated weights, and diversified his workouts. The result? Weight loss, boundless energy, and daily morning bowel movements.

9

Hydration

Do the Unbelievers not realize that the heavens and earth were 'once' one mass then We split them apart? And We created from water every living thing? Will they not then believe?
Al-Anbiya 30

Just as skin cells and organs need liquids to stay hydrated, so does your gut microbiome, as fluid affects how the microbes function and how food is digested and moves through the digestive system — critical aspects of gut health.

Water helps to add moisture and soften stool, thereby keeping food moving through the digestive system and not negatively impacting the microbiome. Water is one of the best ways to stay hydrated, and it is always recommended that you use filtered water to prevent added chemicals from hurting the microbes in your gut.

Certain drinks, such as soft drinks and juices, only feed the bad bacteria in your gut, leading to increased inflammation and weight gain. However, fermented drinks, such as kombucha and kefir, are extremely good for the gut as they provide nutrients while increasing the diversity of microbes. Herbal teas can help feed the good gut microbiome and also help to keep the GI tract moving. Choose drinks that are low in sugar.

If you are unsure how hydrated you are, spend a week or two keeping track of how much liquid you consume in a day. The longer you keep up the tracking, the more accurate a picture you will get.

As you consume liquid throughout the day (outside of Ramadan), be sure that you try to drink a few sips every twenty to thirty minutes to keep your gut healthy and keep the digestive tract moving.

SARAH'S STORY

Sarah came to me struggling with chronic constipation and low energy. We sat down together and began to take a closer look at her diet and lifestyle. We were well into the discussion when I brought up the subject of fluid intake. After pausing momentarily, Sarah admitted that perhaps in a day, she had between one and one and a half cups of water. But she never considered it a problem; after all, she drank a lot of tea—caffeinated tea. Unfortunately, the caffeinated drinks left her with a negative water balance at the end of the day. It was no surprise that she was constipated and had very little energy. Over the next few weeks, we slowly increased her water consumption and added more vegetables to her diet. As we made progress, so did her energy levels, and her bowel movements became more regular.

10

Putting It All Together

Now that you have an idea about why gut health is important and the basics of what negatively and positively affects it, it's time to take a look at yourself and your stress and sleep, your food, your environment, and your activity. As you prepare for the upcoming Ramadan, be sure to look carefully at your overall health.

Ask yourself questions such as:

- How am I feeling today? Do I feel better than I did last year? Or worse?

- What are five things that could negatively be affecting my health?

- What are five changes I can make today to start improving my (gut) health?

- What can I plan on changing in the near future?

It's time to improve your gut's health. You don't need to do a complete 180 on your life today, but start small and keep building upon it, and in no time, you will start feeling and noticing the difference.

It is our responsibility to take care of what has been given to us, including our body and health. It is a gift we must not take for granted.

As the Prophet (*May Peace and Blessings Be Upon Him*) said, 'Indeed, your own self has rights over you' [Abu Dawud]

When you care for your gut's health, you can enjoy a healthy body. Benefits include:

- **An improved digestive system which is critical for nutrient absorption in addition to nutrient digestion and nutrient storage.**

- **A stronger immune system** to increase our resistance against common colds and bugs and deadly strains of diseases and infections. It also promotes quicker healing of cuts and bruises.

- **Improved mental health and moods** as the link between the gut and the brain is incredibly powerful; maintaining a healthy microbiome improves your mental health, focus, concentration, and overall stability.

- **Decrease in inflammation** and better regulation of any inflammation you may have, along with chronic inflammation conditions such as arthritis, obesity, and asthma.

- **Improving your weight and the ability to flush out toxins from your body.**

- **Better skin** and a decrease in symptoms of conditions such as psoriasis, acne, and eczema

- **Less fluctuation in blood sugar** and reducing your risk of diabetes, obesity, and insulin resistance.

- **Improved heart health, reduced allergies and symptoms, improved sleep, improved hormonal balances, and increased energy levels.**

Now is the time to take action for your gut, health, and body. So start today.

Now, let's get into Ramadan!

11

Optimizing Ramadan With Gut Health

Ramadan can be a fantastic month if we choose to get the most out of it. Now, how do we decide to do this, you ask? Start by eating simple, wholesome gut friendly foods.

Always try to avoid things that do not make us feel well, including foods that may give us short-term pleasure because, in the long term, they will cause some sort of damage.

Second, be organized. Ramadan can be a busy month, and if you go into the month thinking that you will miraculously think of what to make an hour before *iftar* time, chances are you will either be stressed out for half that time, or you will end up eating out. Neither of which is good for your gut health.

And third, make the intention to improve your health for the sake of Allah. Our bodies are an *Amanah*, and it is our responsibility to take care of them. Our reward is based on our intention. We are blessed with the ability to change our intention for anything positive and halal that we do in order to gain reward for it. Don't let this opportunity pass you by. Intend to improve or maintain your health for Allah's sake so you can have the energy to worship Him as He intended and so you can take care of and provide for your family.

Lastly, practice gratitude. Allah says, ***If you tried to count God's blessings, you would never be able to number them. Surely God is All-Forgiving, Most Merciful. An-Nahl 18***

There are so many *ayahs* in the Quran and *hadiths* that remind us to be thankful to Allah. Not only is this spiritually rewarding, but it is also beneficial in many other aspects of life that have been scientifically proven.

- Gratitude improves physical health - grateful people observe fewer aches and pains and report feeling healthier than others.

- It also improves psychological health. It reduces toxic emotions, from envy and resentment to frustration and regret.

- Gratitude enhances empathy and reduces aggression.

- Grateful people sleep better.

- Gratitude increases self-esteem.

Taking time every day to either mentally reflect on all your blessings or make a gratitude journal can significantly improve the quality of your life, preparing you for a gut-healthy Ramadan.

Getting Organized

So how do we begin? The first step is to make a meal plan and a grocery list. The best part about this is that once you have a healthy and gut friendly plan, you can use it on repeat for years to come and tweak it as your tastes may change.

Start by asking yourself a few questions, such as:

- What meals do I have to cook?

- Will I have anyone to cook for?

- What are a few must-have dishes that I will cook?

Your answers can be as detailed or as basic as you need them to be. For some, just making a list of dinners and *suhoors* (pre-dawn meals), in no particular order, that will be eaten that week will be enough. You can choose what you make on the day depending on mood and time. For others, it would be worthwhile to get detailed—every meal, for every day.

This may seem like a lot of work, but it will make our weekly planning and shopping much easier and less stressful. If we organize our food so we spend less time and energy on it, we'll have more time for the important things, like *salah*, *dua*, Quran, and *sadaqah*, and overall become more productive.

After making your meal plan, the next step is to make a grocery list and only buy what is on the list. If you are worried about not having enough at a meal, have a few extra freezer items or canned foods (BPA free) like beans on hand that can easily be added to a meal to make it go further. Buying extras of whatever you want can lead to wasting or overeating, neither of which we want to do in Ramadan or outside.

Eat and drink, but do not waste. Surely He does not like the wasteful. Al-Araf 31

Next comes the meal prep. This I highly recommend. Take an hour or two on the weekend and prepare some things you may use often. Personally, I like to spend a few hours before Ramadan and fry up pounds of onions and many heads of garlic, which usually lasts me all of Ramadan.

I chop the onions, fry them until soft, and then add the chopped garlic. Once it's all a nice brown color, I will blend them in a high-speed blender. Then, I'll freeze the mixture in molds. I also blend peeled ginger with water and freeze it in individual molds. Later, I simply take a piece out when needed. This cuts down on time and doesn't cause the house to smell too strongly of cooking smells daily, except on the day you actually do all of this prep!

Other ways to meal prep include chopping up vegetables that you commonly use, at the beginning of the week. This could be onions, carrots, celery, and even cucumbers. Or you could batch cook, which means you cook many portions of a meal and freeze them in meal-size portions so you do not need to cook every day. Choose whatever works for you to cut back on cooking time and possible stress. You can also opt to cook breakfast or dinner casseroles, soups, and one-pot meals well before and freeze them so that when the time comes, all you need to do is defrost and heat! Having three to four freezer meals at all times can be very beneficial to keeping you on track to maintain good health and stop you from turning to unhealthy and fast food options when time gets away from you.

Then, make a list of what you want to accomplish every day, stick to it, and enjoy checking each thing off throughout the day! Having pretty stationary for meal planning or grocery shopping can make the event and planning much more delightful!

When you go grocery shopping, always have your list and stick to it. If you are unaccustomed to sticking to a list, the first few times may be difficult, but view it as another act of self-control and a willingness to change your life. Always shop after a meal so you aren't tempted to buy unneeded food that may ultimately be wasted.

12

Don'ts - Foods to Avoid

Listed on the following pages are foods we should avoid and others we should aim to eat. Remember, everyone is different. What makes one feel good may not necessarily work for another. For example, one person may feel great after eating lentils, and someone else, not so much. So listen to your body and adjust accordingly. Try to keep a food journal. This will help you to pinpoint what could be causing you damage. Mark down everything you eat and drink, your bowel movements, any pain, your physical activity, and your mood. After some time, you'll be able to connect the dots and remove what doesn't work for you. While there will be discrepancies on the same good foods working for everyone, there is mostly consensus on what is harmful for everyone.

If you fall off the wagon, it doesn't mean you stay down. Everyone will have a day or more where, for one reason or another, they ate things that they shouldn't have. When you fall off, get right back on and try again. Go for an extra walk and try to encourage yourself that it was just a slip and not a permanent wrong turn. Don't make it worse by giving up. Keep trying!

It will also be helpful to change your lifestyle and promote gut-healthy living with friends and family. Having a group of people with the same values will help encourage you and maintain the lifestyle for years to come.

Foods to Avoid

"Take advantage of five before five: your youth before your old age, your health before your sickness, your wealth before your poverty, your free time before your busyness, and your life before your death." - Prophet Muhammad (May Peace and Blessings Be Upon him)

What foods should you be avoiding?

1) Sugar

We already mentioned that sugar is highly addicting. On top of that, sugars, especially processed sugars, are damaging to your gut health. Sugar causes bad gut bacteria to flourish and good bacteria to diminish, which can lead to sugar cravings and gut damage. It also makes our blood sugar levels go on a roller coaster ride, unnecessarily activating our cortisol (stress hormones) levels. Our adrenaline levels also peak and crash. In other words, sugar activates hormones that should not be so easily triggered. All this results in cravings, mood swings, depression, poor concentration, poor memory, drops in energy, brain fog, irritability, fatigue, and more. Not the ideal symptoms for Ramadan! Sugar is also a major cause of inflammation in our bodies. Inflammation can be silent in the body, meaning damage is being done, but you don't necessarily feel it until it manifests itself and it usually manifests itself in the form of disease. Avoid sugar as much as possible!

When we say sugar, I don't only mean the white, sweet-tasting thing. I am also referring to foods with a high glycemic index: foods that quickly turn into sugar in the body, i.e., refined flour, wheat bread, white rice, and very starchy vegetables like white potatoes. Aim for foods with a low glycemic index. To find out what the glycemic index is for certain foods, do an internet search for the 'glycemic index food list.'

If you are having a sugar craving, reach for dates! Dates are an excellent source of fiber, vitamins, minerals, and energy. And if your food has added sugar like maple syrup, raw honey, and coconut sugar, which are the better sugars (not white or cane sugar), then pair it with low glycemic foods to reduce the glycemic load or total amount of sugars.

2) Fried Foods

Unfortunately, Ramadan has become the festival of eating, with fried foods being the ultimate fare that represents Ramadan. In some households, *iftars* are not seen as complete if *samosas* and *pakoras* aren't present. Indulging occasionally can be acceptable, but consuming them often is not. Perhaps if people knew the effects of fried foods on our bodies, we would think twice before picking up that oily treat.

So what do fried foods do?

Fried foods make us feel bloated, sluggish, and unable to attain the most from our nighttime prayers. They can also lead to excessive gas and diarrhea and cause harmful bacteria to thrive. They cause inflammation in the body, and as we mentioned, inflammation is the cause of all diseases. They cause excessive, unhealthy weight gain. They clog arteries and veins, which can lead to heart attacks and strokes, amongst other problems. They affect much more than just our gut; they damage nearly every organ and system in our body!

So, how much fried food are you consuming? If you can't give them all up, reduce as much as possible. If you are having multiple pieces every day, reduce to one piece a day. If you have one piece a day, try reducing it to only the weekends. Another option is to cut your portions in half. And if you can drop them altogether, please do so. Switch to baking or air-frying. Your body will thank you for it.

3) Refined flours & Grains

The reason we avoid refined flour and refined grains goes back to the same reasons for sugar. They quickly turn into sugar in our bodies and send us on a roller coaster ride, which usually results in a crash. Not very pleasant! So, choose whole grains. And if you will still have something like white rice, keep your rice portion small and again pair it with lower glycemic foods such as vegetables and protein.

Refined flours are also heavily processed and may contain various chemicals — all damaging to the gut microbiota. Choose organic when possible.

4) Gluten

The modern wheat we eat today is not what our Prophet Muhammad *(May Peace and Blessings Be Upon Him)* ate or even what our ancestors and grandparents ate. It is a hybridized variety with more gluten and significantly fewer nutrients than ancient wheat.

Gluten, present in wheat, barley, rye, and a few other less common grains, has been shown to cause gut damage to most individuals, though the severity and healing varies from person to person. Remember, 70% of our immune system is in our gut, so if we have a damaged or leaky gut, we have a weakened immune system, which leads to all sorts of illnesses.

More immediately, gluten can lead to gas, bloating, discomfort, and possibly diarrhea, and makes it difficult to last a day of fasting. Speaking from experience, when you ditch the gluten-filled *paratha*s and *rotis* (flatbreads) at *suhoor*, you suddenly realize that feeling awful after *suhoor* is not normal! *Suhoor* should be beneficial for your body, and if it doesn't feel like it is, then you must rethink what you are consuming.

On top of that, gluten-containing foods (bread, pasta, etc.) also cause carb cravings, which is the last thing you need when you are fasting. By removing gluten from your diet, you are not missing out on any vital nutrients. You are better off eating other, more nutritious grains.

* What if I can't give up certain ingredients?

Take wheat, for example: what should I do? Choose better-for-you wheat products. Choose items with the least amount of ingredients. Look for sprouted grains, or organic products, and ancient grains. Choose products without added sugar. Even though you are still consuming gluten, it will not have as profound of a negative effect as if you were eating something like Wonder Bread, which doesn't do anything wonderful for gut health. Any change, no matter how small it is, will have a positive effect on your body. Start where you can and keep going.

5) Conventional Cow's Milk

Once milk has been pasteurized, it loses its nutritional value and can become harmful in many ways. It is often the cause of gas, bloating, and diarrhea for many people. While yogurt, kefir, and other dairy forms may benefit some, others may benefit from completely removing dairy from their diet. So listen to your body; only consume dairy if it makes you feel good.

If you are not ready to remove milk from your diet, then only consume organic, so you avoid unnecessary antibiotics and chemical contaminants, or choose raw milk (which has all of its vitamins and minerals) if it is legal where you live.

6) Processed Foods

Foods that come in boxes and cans with tens of unpronounceable ingredients are not really food. To quote Dr. Alejandro Junger, *"The problem is that we are not eating food anymore; we are eating food-like products."* If something has an extremely long shelf life or doesn't decay, chances are it isn't real food. And what do I mean by that? You may be able to eat it; it may taste good and in some cases, deceptively good, but it is devoid of any nutrients. Basically, it is junk or a chemical concoction posing as food that only harms. Remember, real food doesn't have ingredients; it is an ingredient.

For convenience's sake, if you still want processed food occasionally, choose ones with minimal ingredients that do not contain preservatives, artificial colors, sugars, and flavors.

When you shop for food, be mindful of the labeling and marketing that goes into products. Also, be sure to read the ingredient list, double-checking any ingredients you are unfamiliar with.

Even when shopping in the 'health food' aisle, be very careful, as marketing and branding of those products have at times been shown to be very deceptive and no healthier than comparable brand name products.

7) Caffeine

Most caffeine sources are diuretics, meaning they make you eliminate more water or urine than when drinking a non-caffeinated beverage. For one cup of coffee, you need about two additional cups of water to compensate for the lost water. Especially in Ramadan's long, hot days, we do not want to lose more water than we need to. This can lead to dehydration and constipation. But if you have a good relationship with caffeine and want to continue with it, make sure you are getting that extra water in.

8) GMOs

GMOs or Genetically Modified Organisms are organisms that have been altered in a way that does not occur naturally. They are created in laboratories, and their purpose is to introduce specific traits that are not naturally occurring. For example, their primary purpose is to make the plants pest-resistant. Essentially, that means that when a pest, like an insect, bites into the plant, its stomach explodes. If that is what is happening to a pest, what is happening to us? GMOs cause gut damage in humans and animals and are best avoided. Know what items are most often grown as GMOs. That would be corn, soy, sugar beets, summer squash, pink pineapple, and some varieties of apples. To avoid them, look for the Non-GMO label or choose organic when buying these fruits and vegetables or products with them in them. Organic produce cannot be genetically modified.

Also note that GMOs are often fed to animals in factory farms, which is a mass-production farming method that results in sick animals. It's best to choose organic or local, small, farm-raised animals if possible.

13

Do's - What To Eat & Drink

"O believers, eat from the good (Tayyib) things We have provided for you. And give thanks to God if you 'truly' worship Him 'alone.' Al-Baqarah 172

If we want to eat according to Islamic traditions, we must eat *halal* and *Tayyib* foods. *Tayyib* means good, pure, clean, wholesome, gentle, fair and lawful; so basically, anything good, pure, and harmless.

1) Water

Our bodies are made up of around 70% water. If you are feeling thirsty, it means you are already dehydrated. Being dehydrated is often confused with hunger and leads to unnecessary eating. Dehydration causes constipation, abdominal pains, and cramps. It also leads to fatigue, brain fog, depression, anxiety, and muscle weakness, among other symptoms. Water is needed for all systems of the body, especially the brain, so make sure you drink plenty of water at *iftar, suhoor,* and in between. As discussed earlier, water is also critical for your gut health.

Herbal teas, bone broth, lemon, or fruit-infused water will all count toward your water intake. But *Rooh Afza*, soda, and juice are not considered water! So please avoid them.

When choosing teas, you can be intentional in selecting teas that are known to promote a healthy gut. These include:

- Chamomile tea, which contains antioxidants (great for cell repair and a preventative), relaxes GI tract muscles and improves sleep.

- Dandelion root tea, which promotes detoxification of toxins, particularly environmental toxins.

- Fennel tea, which can help prevent or reduce flatulence and bloating, all while reducing discomfort in the GI tract.

- Green tea, which contains minerals and compounds critical for gut health.

- Ginger Root tea, which helps to ease discomfort in the digestive system and is anti-inflammatory.

- Peppermint tea, which helps to relax muscles in the GI tract (helps to move food along) and reduce bloating.

- Turmeric tea, which reduces gut and GI tract inflammation and promotes overall health throughout the system.

2) High Fiber Foods

Most people do not eat enough fiber! Foods that are complex carbohydrates contain fiber. Fiber slows down the absorption of foods, which means it goes through your system slowly, leaving you fuller for longer. As a result, your body will have sustained energy levels and fewer blood sugar swings. Fiber also adds bulk to your stools, promoting regular bowel movements and preventing constipation.

Examples of high-fiber foods are:

- non-starchy vegetables like cruciferous vegetables (broccoli, cauliflower, cabbage, Brussels sprouts, etc.), celery, cucumber, rutabaga, radishes, and peppers

- leafy greens like kale, collard greens, and spinach

- beans and lentils*

- low glycemic fruit like berries**

- whole grains such as millet, oats, amaranth, quinoa, brown rice, sorghum, teff

- chia seeds (add into your smoothies or sprinkle on granola)

Remember to soak your beans, lentils, and grains beforehand to increase their digestibility and prevent gas and bloating.

**Choose organic berries when possible since conventional berries are heavily sprayed with pesticides.*

3) Protein

Proteins are crucial to our bodies functioning properly, particularly on a cellular level. Our blood is made of protein. Our immune health, nervous system, our ability to repair and recover depend on protein. And much of how it all functions depends on how we sleep, making the two aspects uniquely connected and critical to our health.

When many Muslims think of protein, they automatically think of meat. While eating meat is allowed and a *sunnah*, it does not mean we should overindulge or have it with every single meal. The Prophet Muhammad

(May Peace and Blessings Be Upon Him) ate meat, but rarely; sometimes, it would be once a month. So try mixing it up with other forms of protein. Examples of proteins are:

- clean, preferably organic animal meat, and organ meat (avoid factory-farmed animals if possible)

- free range eggs

- wild fish

- sprouts

- seeds, hemp seeds

- nuts

- beans and lentils

- leafy greens and sea vegetables such as kelp, nori, dulse, kombu, and arame

- high-protein foods that people often forget about include cottage cheese and Greek yogurt (if you can tolerate dairy products)

4) Fats

Remember, healthy fats don't make you fat! Our brains are approximately 60% fat, so eating the right fats positively influences your brain. We want to eat unprocessed saturated fats, not the ones in processed foods like margarine. We also want to avoid vegetable, canola, soy, or other highly processed oils. We want them from:

- organic animals
- avocados, avocado oil
- coconut oil, coconut milk, coconut butter, and dried coconut
- raw nuts
- organic butter or ghee
- free-range eggs

Consuming these foods with your meals slows absorption, making you feel satiated for longer. They also help you to absorb fat-soluble vitamins and minerals needed for your body to function properly.

We also want to consume some mono-saturated fats such as:

- olive oil
- avocados
- pumpkin seeds
- sesame seeds

High-quality omega 3s either from:

- Wild salmon
- Walnuts
- Flaxseed
- or a high-quality supplement.

These nutrients will positively assist your mental health.

Some gut conditions, such as inflammatory bowel disease, are directly linked to inflammation in the gut, making it critically important to eat healthy fatty foods as they reduce inflammation.

They also improve the diversity of bacteria in the gut while still feeding and promoting the growth of gut bacteria. This is because many nutrients require fat to absorb particular vitamins, known as fat-soluble vitamins, which are vital for your gut and overall health. Next, healthy fats help keep the walls of your intestines tight to prevent conditions such as leaky gut.

A combination of protein, fats, and fiber with enough water is the best route to staying satiated, hydrated and having a steady flow of energy throughout the day.

5) Fermented Foods

Fermented foods are filled with gut-friendly probiotics that will help your good bacteria proliferate, aid in digestion, and give you a stronger immune system while also promoting heart and mental health. Add a little:

- sauerkraut, kimchi, or fermented pickles to your meals
- some kefir or kombucha
- apple cider vinegar to some warm water to drink at *suhoor* or add some into your salad dressing

Taking a probiotic or a digestive enzyme in supplement form can also boost your digestion.

6) Prophetic & Quranic Foods

It's a good idea to incorporate some Sunnah foods that the Prophet (*May Peace and Blessings Be Upon Him*) ate or Quranic foods mentioned in the Quran. Each and every one of them is nutritious and loaded with vitamins and minerals with different health benefits. By making the intention to eat these foods because they are Prophetic or Quranic foods, gives you the added benefit of receiving a reward from Allah.

Fruits and vegetables:

- Dates
- Grapes
- Pomegranate
- Watermelon
- Olives
- Cucumber
- Squash & pumpkin
- Onions
- Chards
- Mushrooms
- Garlic
- Herbs

Proteins:

- Poultry
- Meat
- Organ meat
- Fish
- Broth
- Lentils

Other:

- Black Seeds
- Honey
- Vinegar
- Olive oil

Feel free to add in some fruit salad with some Sunnah and Quranic foods for a light, refreshing treat after *Maghrib* that can give you a good burst of energy to help you get through your night prayers. And, of course, eat some dates; it's a *sunnah* to break your fast with them and an excellent source of fiber and energy.

What else?

Remember, variety is key to good health. You do not want to eat the same things every day. By mixing it up, you reduce your chances of chronic diseases. Nutrient deficiencies can lead to disease. Add in a diverse amount of vegetables, fruits, grains, proteins, and fats to ensure you are ingesting as many vitamins and minerals as possible to avoid nutrient deficiencies. And do not be afraid of spices. There is a misconception out there that if a food tastes good, it can't possibly be healthy. This is completely false. Almost all spices have medicinal benefits. I'm not talking about packaged spice mixes with preservatives and other additives, but pure, preferably organic spices. Spices can fight inflammation, reduce blood sugar, improve memory function, reduce nausea, boost immunity, and so much more. So add in some spices and some sea salt or Himalayan pink salt (avoid table salt). Eating healthy can definitely taste good!

14

AVOID OVEREATING

Remember, our **Prophet Muhammad, *(May Peace and Blessings be Upon Him)*** said: *"No human ever filled a vessel worse than the stomach. Sufficient for any son of Adam are some morsels to keep his back straight. But if it must be, then one-third for his food, one-third for his drink, and one-third for his breath."* [*Ahmad, At-Tirmidhi, An-Nasaa'I, Ibn Majah - Hadith sahih*].

This is the reason why I wanted to write on this topic originally. Several years ago, I came across an embarrassing article about Muslims in a Muslim-majority country being hospitalized during Ramadan for overeating! Unfortunately, so many of our Muslim brothers and sisters overeat and do precisely the opposite of what our Prophet *(May Peace and Blessings be Upon Him)* advised.

Overeating causes drowsiness, digestive distress, unnecessary weight gain, and wastefulness.

So eat what you need and don't overeat. At the time of iftar, I recommend breaking your fast with dates and a glass of water. Then, after praying maghrib, have your meal. The water from *iftar* should have filled you a bit and will help prevent overeating. For dinner, I suggest using a lunch-sized plate. Often, we like to eat with our eyes and fill our plates. Using a smaller plate will ensure a smaller portion.

Usually, that first helping is enough to satisfy and nourish you. Taking seconds often leads to overeating and regret. Slow down, chew your food repeatedly, and take your time eating. Increasing your chewing and having conversation during your meal allows the digestive juices to flow and promote more efficient digestion; this way, you will extract many more nutrients from your food. Sometimes, we eat so fast that we don't give our brain enough time to process that we've eaten enough until it's too late; by then, we will have already overeaten. We really do not need as much food as we think we do!

Final Thoughts

Plan ahead so there is less stress, time, and energy put into cooking so you can focus on more important things! Listen to your body to learn its likes and dislikes. Remove the junk foods that cause inflammation and bloating, and avoid overeating so that during periods of long *rukhoos* and *sujoods*, you aren't struggling to breathe but are connecting with your Creator. Choose a nutrient-dense combination of protein, fats, and fiber so you have the energy to get through the day, and to be able to worship at night. Improve your sleep, reduce your stress and toxin load, and work on your physical activity to get the best gut health possible in time for Ramadan and the rest of the year!

May Allah make it easy for us all and make it our best Ramadan yet, *Ameen*! If this was of any benefit to you, please remember me and my family in your *duas*, and please consider leaving me a review on the platform you purchased this on.

Bonus recipes on the following pages to give you inspiration for *suhoor* and *iftar*!

Just for readers of my book, join my email list and get a free Ramadan Meal Plan with over 35 healthy and tasty recipes!

www.wellnessreclaimed.com/ramadanguide

Bonus Recipes

Enjoy these Ramadan recipes. Adjust spices to your taste and use them as inspiration!

Chocolate Smoothie with Avocado

Servings: 2 Prep time: 7 min

Ingredients:

- 1 avocado
- 2 cups non-dairy milk
- 2 tbsp nut/seed butter of choice
- 2 cups baby spinach or baby kale
- 1/4 cup chocolate protein powder
- optional: 1/4 cup collagen powder

Directions:

Place all ingredients in a high speed blender. Blend until smooth. Enjoy!

Egg on Sweet Potato with Avocado

Servings: 2 Prep time: 10 min Cook time: 10 min

Ingredients:

- 1 wide sweet potato
- 4 eggs
- 1 avocado
- sea salt or Himalayan pink salt to taste
- black pepper to taste

Directions:

1. Cut the ends off of the sweet potato. Cut sweet potato lengthwise into 1/4 inch slices. You will want 4 pieces. Save any leftovers for another day by storing in an airtight container.

2. Put sweet potato slices into a toaster and toast 2-3x until cooked (soft but not mushy).

3. While the sweet potato cooks, remove the avocado fruit from the peel and place it in a bowl, mash, and season with salt and pepper.

4. Fry eggs in butter or coconut/avocado oil or hard-boil your eggs.

5. Spread mashed avocado on each sweet potato and top with an egg. Season with salt and pepper, and enjoy!

Overnight Oats

Servings: 2 Prep time: 5 min Set time: 4-8 hours

Ingredients:

- 1 cup rolled oats
- 1.5 cups non-dairy milk
- 1/2 cup diced apples
- 2 tbsp chopped walnuts
- 2 tbsps chia seeds
- 2 tbsps maple syrup
- optional: 1/2 cup full fat greek yogurt (if chosen, reduce milk by 1/2 cup)

Directions:

Combine oats, milk, chia seeds, maple syrup, and Greek yogurt (if chosen). Mix in a bowl and then divide it into single serve jars. Top with apples and walnuts. Refrigerate for four to eight hours before eating. Enjoy!

Chickpea & Tuna Salad

Servings: 4Prep time: 15 min

Ingredients:

- 2 cups chickpeas cooked
- 1 can of tuna drained
- 4 green onion stalks chopped
- 1 cup baby spinach chopped
- 1/2 cup cilantro or parsley chopped
- 1/4 cup olive oil
- 1 lemon juiced (or 2 limes)
- sea salt or pink salt to taste
- black pepper to taste

Directions:

1. Combine the chickpeas, tuna, green onions, baby spinach, cilantro or parsley in a large bowl.

2. In a small bowl combine olive oil, lemon juice, salt, and pepper.

3. Add the dressing to the chickpea mixture. Mix.

4. Taste and add more lemon or salt if needed. Enjoy!

Cauliflower Lentil Soup

Servings: 4 Prep time: 15 min Cook time: 40 min

Ingredients:

- 2 tbsps coconut oil or avocado oil
- 1 onion chopped
- 4 garlic cloves finely chopped
- 1 knob of ginger grated
- 3 carrots peeled and chopped
- 3 stalks of celery chopped
- 2 cups of baby spinach or baby kale
- 1 head of cauliflower chopped into florets
- 1 cup of brown lentils (soaked for four hours or more)
- 5 cups of broth (good quality bullion can be used)
- sea salt or pink salt to taste

- black pepper to taste
- 1 tsp turmeric
- 1 tsp cumin powder
- 1 tsp coriander powder
- optional: 1 tsp crushed chilies

Directions:

1. In a large pot, heat oil on medium. Add in onions and saute for three minutes. Add in garlic, ginger, carrots, and celery. Saute for the more minutes.

2. Add in spices and cook for one minute.

3. Add in broth and lentils and cook covered for 20 minutes.

4. Add in cauliflower and spinach and cook for about 15-20 minutes or until the lentils are soft. Add in more water if you want a thinner consistency. Bring back to a boil.

5. Season with salt and pepper to taste. Enjoy!

Mongolian Beef

Instant Pot Recipe

Servings: 5 Prep time: 10 min Cook time: 30 min

Ingredients:

- 2 tbsp coconut oil or avocado oil
- 1 knob of ginger grated
- 5 garlic cloves minced
- 1 lb flank steak thinly cut
- 1/2 cup Braggs soy seasoning
- 4 cups broccoli florets
- 2 carrots sliced or julienne
- 1 cup water divided
- 1/4 cup coconut sugar
- 2 tbsp arrowroot powder*
- 2 stalks green onion thinly sliced
- 1/2 cup cilantro chopped
- 1 tsp chili flakes (optional)
- 1/2 tsp black pepper (optional)

Directions:

1. In an instant pot, turn on the saute function. Add in the coconut oil and when heated add in the garlic and ginger. Mix

and cook for a minute.

2. Then add in the beef and cook until the meat has browned.

3. Now, add in the soy seasoning, coconut sugar, crushed chilies, and black pepper. Mix well.

4. Add in 1/2 cup water and mix well. Turn off the saute function. Put the lid on the sealing position. Press 'manual' or the pressure button and set the time for 12 minutes.

5. When time is up, release the pressure, open the lid and push the off button, and then turn the saute function back on.

6. Add in carrots and cook for three minutes. Then add in the broccoli and cook until slightly tender.

7. Mix 1/2 cup of cool water with the arrowroot powder in a cup. Add the arrowroot/water mixture into the pot and mix. The sauce will thicken at this point. Add more water if you would like a thinner consistency. Or add more arrowroot/water if you would like it thicker.

8. Turn off the instant pot. Top with green onions and cilantro and serve with brown rice or quinoa or something else of your choice. Enjoy!

* Can be substituted with tapioca powder.

Gluten Free Roti

Servings: 2 Prep: 5 min Cook time: 30 min

Ingredients:

- 1/2 cup sorghum flour
- 1/2 cup cassava flour
- 1.5 tsp psyllium husk
- 2 pinches sea salt
- 1 tbsp avocado oil (or coconut oil plus more for step 5)
- 2/3 cup warm water (plus a little more if needed)

Directions:

1. Combine all dry ingredients in a medium sized bowl.

2. Add in warm water and oil, and mix by hand. If necessary add in more warm water, one tablespoon at a time until a soft dough is formed. It should not be sticky, but it should not be dry either.

3. Let the dough sit covered for 30 minutes.

4. If using a tortilla press, divide the dough into 6 pieces. If using a rolling pin, either 6 or 4 will work. Roll or flatten out using parchment paper.

5. Heat pan on medium heat. When the pan is heated, place one flattened circle on the pan. Flip after one minute. After about

30 seconds place a dime sized amount of oil or butter and then flip again. The roti will soon start to puff again and you can flatten it with a spatula. After about 30 seconds flip again. Cook for about 30 seconds more, then you can remove it from the heat. Enjoy!

Ginger Lemonade with Aloe

Servings: 2 Prep time: 5 min Cook time: 15 min

Ingredients:

- 1 knob of ginger peeled

- 2.5 cups of water

- 4 tbsp lemon juice

- 2 tbsp maple syrup

- 1/4 cup pure aloe juice

Directions:

1. Add water to a small saucepan and bring to boil. Add in ginger and cover. Bring heat down to medium low and let it boil for 15 minutes.

2. Remove the pan from heat and allow it to come down to room

temperature.

3. Add in lemon juice, maple syrup, and aloe. Mix well.

4. Add into serving glasses with ice. Enjoy!

Glossary

alhamdulilah - All praise is to Allah

amanah - a trust

ameen - May it be fulfilled

ayah – a verse in the Quran

cytokines - proteins that are vital to communication and signaling between cells

dhikr - remembrance of Allah

dua - a supplication

hadith – a report of sayings or doings attributed to the Prophet Muhammad (*May Peace and Blessings Be Upon Him*)

halal - lawful or permitted

Iftar - the meal when breaking the fast

maghrib – the prayer after sunset

pakora – deep fried fritter

pathogen – an organism that causes a disease

paratha - oily flatbread

roti - flatbread

Rooh Afza - sugar sweetened rose syrup used to make drinks

rukhoos - bowing in prayer

sadaqah - charity

salah - Islamic prayer

samosa - a fried pastry with savory filling

suhoor - pre-dawn meal

sujood - prostration

sunnah - the sayings and doings of the Prophet Muhammad (May Peace and Blessings Be Upon Him)

tayyib - halal, pure, lawful

Resources

Mu, Q., Kirby, J., Reilly, C. M., & Luo, X. (2017). Leaky gut as a danger signal for autoimmune diseases. *Frontiers in Immunology*, 8. https://doi.org/10.3389/fimmu.2017.00598

Campos, M., MD. (2023, September 12). *Leaky gut: What is it, and what does it mean for you?* Harvard Health. https://www.health.harvard.edu/blog/leaky-gut-what-is-it-and-what-does-it-mean-for-you-2017092212451#:~:text=Some%20studies%20show%20that%20leaky,obesity%2C%20and%20even%20mental%20illness.

Institute for Quality and Efficiency in Health Care (IQWiG). (2020, July 30). *The innate and adaptive immune systems.* InformedHealth.org - NCBI Bookshelf. https://www.ncbi.nlm.nih.gov/books/NBK279396/

Janeway, C. A., Jr. (2001). *Principles of innate and adaptive immunity.* Immunobiology - NCBI Bookshelf. https://www.ncbi.nlm.nih.gov/books/NBK27090/#:~:text=After%20a%20naive%20lymphocyte%20has,a%20delay%20of%20several%20days.

Your Digestive System & How it Works. (2023, February 28). National Institute of Diabetes and Digestive and Kidney Diseases. https://www.niddk.nih.gov/health-information/digestive-diseases/digestive-system-how-it-works

Bsn, J. C., RN. (2023, February 13). *What Are Obesogens? Endocrineweb.* Retrieved May 14, 2023, from https://www.endocrineweb.com/conditions/obesity/what-are-obesogens

Allan, S. (2023). *How Nutrition Can Support Gut Health and the Immune System.* Canadian Digestive Health Foundation.

Diet and IBD: Fats, inflammation, and the microbiome - News and events - Crohn's and Colitis Canada. (2023, December 20). https://crohnsandcolitis.ca/News-Events/News-Releases/Diet-and-IBD-Fats,-Inflammation,-and-the-Microbiom#:~:text=The%20takeaway%20for%20individuals%20with,%2C%20offers%20essential%20omega%2D3s.

Stress effects on the body. (2023b, March 8). https://www.apa.org. https://www.apa.org/topics/stress/body

Nunez, K. (2020, July 20). *What Is the Purpose of Sleep? Healthline.* https://www.healthline.com/health/why-do-we-sleep#:~:text=Many%20biological%20processes%20happen%20during,molecules%20like%20hormones%20and%20proteins

How Lack Of Sleep Can Affect Gut Health. (n.d.). Henry Ford Health - Detroit, MI. https://www.henryford.com/blog/2021/02/sleep-affects-gut-health#:~:text=Lack%20of%20sleep%20can%20increase%20stress%2C%20which%20affects%20the%20gut.&text=This%20can%20lead%20to%20a,Barish.

Endomune Advanced Probiotics. (2021). *Are Gut-Harming Chemicals Hiding in Your Home? EndoMune Probiotics.* https://endomune.com/household-chemicals-and-gut-health/

Healthspan. (n.d.). Why exercise is good for your digestive system. https://www.healthspan.co.uk/advice/why-exercise-is-good-for-your-digestive-system

Tu, P., Chi, L., Bodnar, W. M., Zhang, Z., Gao, B., Bian, X., Stewart, J. R., Fry, R. C., & Lü, K. (2020). Gut Microbiome toxicity: Connecting the environment and Gut Microbiome-Associated diseases. Toxics, 8(1), 19. https://doi.org/10.3390/toxics8010019

Warner, D. (2023, November 15). Do antibiotics harm healthy gut bacteria? https://www.medicalnewstoday.com/articles/do-antibiotics-harm-healthy-gut-bacteria#:~:text=Antibiotics%20may%20not%20only%20harm,to%20treat%20a%20bacterial%20infection.

McEvoy, B. M. E. (2011, December 12). The putrid Truth about Pasteurized & Homogenized Dairy. Metabolic Healing. https://metabolichealing.com/the-putrid-truth-about-pasteurized-homogenized-dairy/

Lipton, B. (2023, July 27). How gut health impacts sleep (And vice versa). Sleep.com. https://www.sleep.com/sleep-health/how-gut-health-impacts-sleep#:~:text=Good%20sleep%20helps%20the%20gut%20%E2%80%A6&text=%E2%80%9CStudies%20have%20found%20that%20sleep,stress%20hormones%20in%20the%20body.%E2%80%9D

Vanhaecke, T., Bretin, O., Poirel, M., & Tap, J. (2022). Drinking Water Source and Intake Are Associated with Distinct Gut Microbiota Signatures in US and UK Populations. The Journal of Nutrition, 152(1), 171–182. https://doi.org/10.1093/jn/nxab312

Health benefits of gratitude. (n.d.). UCLA Health. https://www.uclahealth.org/news/health-benefits-gratitude

Rd, J. K. M. (2019, March 6). Is gluten bad for you? A critical look. Healthline. https://www.healthline.com/nutrition/is-gluten-bad#safety

The Clear Quran. (n.d.). https://theclearquran.org/

www.ingramcontent.com/pod-product-compliance
Lightning Source LLC
Chambersburg PA
CBHW071724020426
42333CB00017B/2380